TO THE MAX!

How I Went From Being a Fat, Sick and Tired Mess to Living a Life Filled with Success, Happiness, Health and Fulfillment.

And... how you can do it too!

ISBN: 150307966X
ISBN 13: 9781503079663
Library of Congress Control Number: 2014919796
CreateSpace Independent Publishing Platform
North Charleston, South Carolina

FIRST PRINTING

Printed in the USA

For more information:
Visit: themaxchallenge.com
Email: bryan@themaxchallenge.com
Contact: MAX Headquarters
285 Gordons Corner Road
Manalapan, NJ 07726
Call: (732) 536-4797

The most significant lesson that I have learned in my life is that my outward appearance is only a reflection of what is happening on the inside, and that lasting change is only possible when we change from the inside out. I am honored to have this opportunity to share what I have learned with you and hope that your journey towards improved health, happiness and fitness is as exciting as mine!

I look forward to our shared success.

– Bryan

TO THE MAX!

How I Went From Being a Fat, Sick and
Tired Mess to Living a Life Filled with Success,
Happiness, Health and Fulfillment.

And... how you can do it too!

BRYAN KLEIN

A FIVE-STAGE JOURNEY.

Dedication
Lori, Elijah, Ella, Peyton

Contents

My Story

Your Story

My Story

In My Eyes

When it comes to losing weight, it seems everyone wants to know the answer to the infamous question, "How did you do it?" If it were as simple as sitting here and dictating a diet and exercise plan to anyone who asked me that question, no one would have any problems with weight. When thinking about how my transformation came about, a more important question comes to mind. Maybe it is not so much about how I did it… maybe it is about *why* I did it.

When I was at my heaviest weight of 270 pounds, I did not even realize that a change needed to be made. My belief was, **'What good is living life if you are not going to enjoy yourself?'** I truly felt I was living the "good life". I looked at the few people I knew who followed a more nutritious lifestyle and thought, 'Look at these **fools**. They are depriving themselves of all the fun and food that life has to offer.' I did not realize it at the time, but looking back I can see that *I* was the fool! I was the one depriving myself of reaching my full potential, of enjoying my kids and of experiencing a great many things that life has to offer. Even worse, I was shortening my potential lifespan and practically ensuring a long, drawn out, horrible death at the hands of heart disease, cancer, diabetes or any of the other myriad obesity-related diseases.

Now that I am within my healthy weight range, an entire world of opportunity has opened up to me. I have tried countless things that I would never have had the confidence or the ability to do before. I have completed the Ultimate Black Belt Test, backpacked the Sierra Nevada Mountains and raced in a half-marathon. I even fought in a full contact kickboxing bout. If I were still 270 pounds, I would have cheated myself out of all of these experiences. But more importantly, I would have cheated myself out of all of the *true* daily pleasures – such as enjoying spending time with my family, running down the street after my kids or walking through a park without getting exhausted; the list goes on and on.

Looking back on my experiences I now realize that I was suffering from something far greater than the "obesity epidemic". I had traded all those possible life-enriching experiences for an unhealthy diet and called it the good life. I was suffering from the even greater threat of the "mediocrity epidemic" and I had become content with living a life void of excellence and passion!

I hope that you can benefit from my journey and the stories I tell throughout this book, and that you too can break free from the chains of your past to not only lose the weight but also live a life of purpose, passion, and fulfillment. Take it to THE MAX!

STAGE 1

Conceive Your Vision

"All successful people men and women are big dreamers. They imagine what their future could be, ideal in every respect, and then they work every day toward their distant vision, that goal or purpose."

– Brian Tracy

CHAPTER 1

New York, New York

The city that never sleeps, filled with bright lights and a skyline that is recognizable around the world, New York City is known as the place where dreams are made. Songs with such empowerment were made famous by legends such as Frank Sinatra; however, the city of New York holds a different significance for me – desperation.

I could not have been happier when I found out that I was going to be a father. I began to hope, imagine and dream of what life would be like as a parent. My wife Lori and I began to make plans for our new child. We would stay up late into the night wondering, will it be a boy or a girl? What will he or she look like? What kind of personality will the new baby have? What will we name him or her? Each of these conversations would end with the same thought, "As long as the baby is healthy, that is all that matters." I can remember that it was an exciting time filled with possibilities and hope.

After about twenty weeks, my wife and I received news from our doctor that would ultimately transform my entire outlook on life. My wife had an amniocentesis performed, a routine test where they make a small hole in the womb to check the baby for genetic abnormalities. Although the puncture is generally supposed to heal quickly, the hole in the sac failed to close, causing fluid to escape. An ultrasound revealed that most of the amniotic fluid had leaked out of the womb. Without this, the baby's lungs could not develop properly. The doctor advised us to immediately terminate the pregnancy. He stressed that if we continued with the pregnancy our child would die, or at best live a life of misery. He finished giving us the news by explaining that by prolonging our decision we were needlessly putting my wife's health at risk and advised us to "get it over with" and "move on". Needless to say my wife was not taking this news well. She broke down in tears as all of her hopes and dreams seemed to be slipping away. I knew I needed to be strong. I took my wife by the hand, let her know that somehow things would work out, and stormed out of the office never to return.

Determined not to give up, I began to look for a solution to our problem. I tried the internet, the library, asking friends, anyone and anything I could think of that might provide some possibility. Then I remembered – one of my students had mentioned that her father was, at one time, the head of Labor and Delivery at NYU Medical Center. She arranged for us to have a conversation on the phone with him and, by the next day, we found ourselves in the office of his associate, Dr. Bruce Young. He gave us several options, including the chance to undergo an experimental procedure that might save our baby and protect my wife. We took him up on the offer immediately.

My wife and unborn son were in surgery the next day. I will never forget the moment when Dr. Young came out of surgery to update us on the procedure. He let me know that, although this was the first time he performed this surgery, he felt confident that we would ultimately have a healthy child. Then he handed me a picture of my growing son's hand that they took during the procedure. Looking back on the situation now, the most significant thing that Dr. Young gave us was hope. Things were settling down for the moment and we were getting prepared to move in to what would be our "home" for more than three months – Room 1314 at New York University Medical Center.

Every day was like a roller coaster ride for the emotions. My wife was connected to machines to constantly monitor her blood pressure and heart rate, and the development of our unborn son was assessed continuously throughout the day. Every beep of the machine or report from the lab brought another, and often contradictory, report. One minute things are stable, the next they are uncertain. One minute everything looks good, then things suddenly change and they would rush my wife into labor and delivery where we would spend hours or days until things would stabilize and we could move back to Room 1314. The stress of the situation constantly changing from safe, to crisis mode, then back to stable was very difficult for us.

One afternoon as the doctor was making his routine visit my nervous energy must finally have become too much for him to deal with. He recommended that I take a walk to unwind as he examined my wife. As I began to explore the neighborhood I quickly realized that there were more restaurants on one block than in our entire town. My mood began to lift a bit as I thought about how exciting it was going to be to try all these new places. My focus quickly went from, 'What the hell is going to happen to my family?' to, 'What the heck am I going to eat today? There are so many great choices!'

I walked out to the corner where was a small pizza shop called "Pizza and Pita". I thought, 'How can this get any better? You can get a pizza and a pita all in one place!' And although the restaurant was small, the pizza slices were huge! I stared over the counter and suddenly the biggest decision I had to make was choosing between the chicken Parmesan, pepperoni and sausage or cheesesteak pizza. I ordered two slices with pepperoni and sausage and sat down at the first available table. I took that first bite and thought, 'Wow, that tastes great!' It seemed that with each and every bite of the pizza my problems were pushed further and further back into my mind. I washed the meal down with a huge tub of Coke and happily made my way back to the hospital.

The next day was not much different. The situation was real again, the stress was back, and so as the doctors made their rounds I "stepped out for a minute". This is how my routine began. As I would walk towards the elevators, I would start to think about the world of possibilities that would open up to me once I reached the ground floor and I began to push my problems further into the back of my mind. For the next three months I would look forward to the doctors' visits to my wife's room because for me it was a chance to discover another of New York's great restaurants. The 2nd Ave Deli, The Great American Grilled Cheese Factory, the Number One Chinese Restaurant, Ess-a-Bagel and "Dirty Water Dogs" from the corner became some of my favorite escapes.

Late one night, the doctor decided to move us to labor and delivery for the last time. They explained that my wife's blood pressure was dangerously high, and that while every day my son spent growing in the womb gave him an increased chance at survival and living a full life, each day also increased the risk to my wife's health. We moved to our new room on the delivery floor and they administered medication to keep Lori's blood pressure down. They told us that they would need to do the delivery any day. My wife could not get out of bed, but they arranged for a counselor to come talk to us about the dangers associated with pre-term delivery and took me on a tour of the NICU (neonatal intensive care unit). To make matters worse, the medication Lori was on was making her feel even more ill. I was extremely strained – if the thought of being a first-time parent was not enough, my child and wife's health were both in question. I was fast approaching an uncertain future. My mind was racing. Would my wife come out of this healthy? Would my child survive? Would he be capable of breathing on his own? What else could I do but take a walk to the 2nd Ave Deli for a corned beef sandwich?

I walked several blocks to make it to the deli where they recognized me as a regular. During my meal all of my worries seemed to disappear. I had a smile on my face. I felt refreshed and was ready for my walk back to my wife's side. As I approached the room I heard the head nurse shout out "Code Blue". I ran into the room to find the nurse and several doctors standing over Lori's bed turning her onto her side. Within seconds the room was filled with the doctors and nurses that had become our friends and family over the past several months. I was instructed to leave the room where, within seconds, they began an emergency Caesarean section. I waited out in the hall hoping and praying that everything would be all right. I looked into the nursery where the healthy babies were and thought, 'Please just let everything turn out okay and I will promise to be the best father and person I can be. I will strive to set the best example I can for my son, students and community and I promise to make a difference for others who are going through similar situations.'

A few minutes later, the nurse invited me in to meet my newborn, two-pound, 12-ounce son – Elijah.

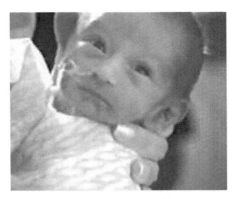

Elijah, a few hours old

I realize now that this was not the beginning of just one new life, but of two new lives. On that day I had conceived a new and exciting vision for the future of my life. A future where I would fulfill my promise to reach my potential – to become the best parent and martial arts instructor that I could be, and to help others through similar situations.

There was only one problem...

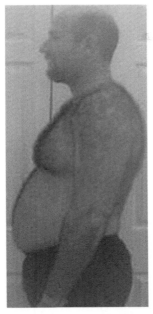

Me, at my maximum weight of 270 pounds

...this is what I looked like!

CHAPTER 2

Fulfilling My Promise

As much as I wanted to achieve my vision, there was something holding me back. Each time that I would start working towards losing weight, I would get distracted and sidetracked. I would join a gym and work out hard for three months – but, when I looked in the mirror, I didn't see a change, so I stopped going to the gym. I set up a training schedule for myself – but after a couple of months I didn't see the results I wanted, so I would stop following it. I knew that in order to make the impact that I wanted for myself, my family, my students and my community I would have to be a role model of excellence. I knew that I would have to get into the best shape of my life. Not only would it be important for the impression that I was making, but also I needed to be capable of focusing for long periods of time so that I could take consistent daily action towards the achievement of my vision.

I could not escape from my vision for a better future. Although I would sometimes lose sight of what I was supposed to be working towards, the promise I made the day my son was born would always come back to me. I began to realize that what I looked like was not really the problem. It was what my physical appearance represented that was holding me back. It was obvious to everyone that I was soft on the outside but what my friends, family and students did not know was that I was soft on the inside as well. It was clear to the naked eye that my body was not in the best shape it could have been, but what was not as obvious was that my outer appearance was only a reflection of all the compromises I was making on the inside. I was settling for being less than I could be – as a parent, a martial artist, a businessperson and as a member of my community. I had become not only a victim of obesity but a victim of mediocrity as well. What was really holding me back was not what I looked like on the outside but how I was feeling on the inside.

I began to realize that if I were ever going to achieve my vision I would need to not only change my physical appearance. I would need to challenge my beliefs and completely reinvent myself from the inside out.

STAGE 2

Challenge Your Beliefs

"Keep your dreams alive. Understand to achieve anything requires faith and belief in yourself, vision, hard work, determination, and dedication. Remember all things are possible for those who believe."

– Gail Devers

CHAPTER 3

Attack of the 'What Ifs'

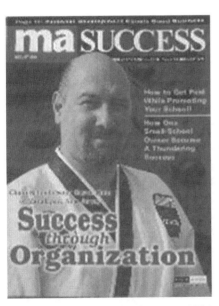

Martial Arts Success Cover, August 2004

In 2004 I was on the cover of the Martial Arts Industry magazine. There was a five-page article titled "The Most Successful Martial Arts School Owner on the East Coast" written about me. It was a great honor, but in time I came to define myself as 'the guy on the magazine cover'. That image on the front of that magazine became the façade that I would hold up to protect myself from how I was really feeling on the inside. I found myself buying things that I did not need in order to support my "image". Fast cars, big houses, expensive clothes... to everyone else I had it all – respect, freedom and all the material fixings. But every time my friends would invite me to some adventure – a hiking trip, a special workout or a martial arts tournament – I would turn down the offer to protect the image of 'the guy on the magazine cover'. I would make excuses to myself; I was too busy growing the schools, too busy with my family, too busy doing whatever the excuse of the day was.

The truth was that I wanted nothing more than to compete in the tournament, participate in the special workout or go on the hike, but I was afraid of what people would think. Would I live up to the image of 'the guy on the magazine cover'? What if I was to compete, and lost? Would my students still respect me? What if I couldn't keep up with the others on the hike? Would my friends lose respect for me? What if I couldn't measure up to the expectations that the others in the class had set for me? What if... what if... what if...?

So I kept telling myself the same story, over and over, until even I started to believe it. 'I don't have time for tournaments... I am too busy being a businessperson.' 'I don't have time for backpacking... I am too busy with my family.' 'I don't have time to train – I am the busy guy on the cover of the magazine.' Each and every one of those lines was just one more compromise that chiseled away at my confidence and belief in myself.

All of the 'what ifs' were holding me back from truly reaching my potential and I was robbing myself of becoming the best martial artist, parent and person I could possibly be. They were ultimately keeping me from fulfilling my vision and promise. Deep down inside I knew that if I was going to achieve my vision I would need to face the truth and finally do battle with the 'what ifs'. I was about to embark on the first step of a life-changing journey towards completely reinventing myself.

CHAPTER 4

A Swift Kick in the Ass!

One event would redirect the course of my life and finally put me on track to make good on my promises. A good friend of mine, Alicia, had just enrolled in a martial arts challenge program called the Ultimate Black Belt Test (UBBT). This test was run by Tom Callos, one of the most respected martial arts masters of our time and one of my own personal heroes. Although I never had the opportunity to meet Tom, he was always someone whom I had studied from a distance and looked towards for inspiration. Alicia invited me to join her in the UBBT. She gave me a list of the requirements and it took me only a few seconds to realize that this was not for me – 'the guy on the magazine cover' façade took over immediately. *Some* of the requirements included:

- 52,000 sit-ups
- 52,000 push-ups
- Journal your daily experiences and meditate daily for a year
- Spar 1,000 rounds
- Perform and record 1,000 Random Acts of Kindness
- Perform a kata (martial arts routine) 1,000 times
- Lead an environmental clean-up program
- Participate in a house-building project in Alabama
- Backpack in the Sierra Nevada mountains
- Participate in the (grueling) final exam

I got to the first line in the list and the all-too-familiar excuses started coming out. 'I don't have time for this. Who would run my school
while I was out doing these activities? My family needs me at home.'
The list went on. Deep inside I wanted nothing more than to participate
in this program and to earn the respect of my peers, seniors, family and
friends, but at the time the 'what ifs' were too strong. The image I had
built of myself, as 'the guy on the magazine cover' was too much to
overcome. Once again I backed down from the invitation for fear that I
could not complete the requirements.

A few months later I came across an advertisement in a martial arts
magazine advertising that Tom Callos was looking for school owners
to host seminars at their schools. I asked Alicia for his phone number
and eventually worked up the courage to give him a call. After a few
minutes of discussion we had made the arrangements for him to travel
to New Jersey to teach a seminar for my students, but in the back of my
mind I knew that his true motive was to enroll me in the Ultimate Black
Belt Test.

I still remember a phone conversation where Tom insisted that whatever hotel I put him up in must have a well-equipped gym. I remember thinking to myself, 'is this guy for real? Are there people who take
themselves so seriously that they do not take a day off from training?' I
was about to find out. The day I picked Tom up at the airport, he got off
the airplane, greeted me with a big hug, and asked, "So have you been
training hard or hardly training?" My mind started racing. 'What if he
asks me to work out with my students? Am I going to be able to keep up
with this guy? I hope he does not think any less of me after this weekend,' There was no need for me to answer his question – my physical
appearance, sweaty forehead and nervous disposition told it all. I took a
deep breath and thought to myself, 'This is going to be a long weekend!'

I assumed I would take Tom to his hotel and check him in, but he had
other plans. "Let's go straight to your dojo and meet your team." We ar-
rived at the school to find our usual Friday instructor class being led by
one of the more senior instructors. Tom found the changing room, threw
on his uniform and began to participate in the class! It wasn't more than
a few minutes before he invited me to join him and the others. As we
started to train I honestly don't know what hurt more at that moment

– the pain my body was feeling from not being used to that level of training, or the emotional pain I was feeling from all the 'what ifs' that were still running through my mind.

The weekend did not get any easier. Tom had me working out in front of and with my students on Friday, Saturday and Sunday. When things seemed like they could not possibly get any worse, in front of almost 100 people he announced that after "much thought and discussion" I had decided to take part in his Ultimate Black Belt Test. I was thinking to myself, 'what the #$^% is he talking about, we didn't discuss any of this!' He continued by saying that they should all be very proud of their instructor for taking on the challenge and began listing all of the seemingly impossible requirements. As he read each one off the list, another bead of sweat would form on head, and another 'what if' would run through my mind. I literally felt sick to my stomach and felt like pooping my pants! Then Tom ended it by saying, "Let's all congratulate your instructor for having the courage to take on a challenge that only a few individuals have completed. Give him a big round of applause and wish him luck!" The room burst out in clapping and cheering. People with looks of tremendous admiration in their eyes were high-fiving me and patting me on the back. I smiled as I looked around the room and thanked everyone for their support, but in my mind I had a vision of me standing in front of Tom giving him the double-handed salute (a gesture passed on to me by my grandfather where you extend both middle fingers into the air and give rapid-fire flip-offs). At the time I hated him for it, but in hindsight Tom did me a huge favor that day... *he gave me the kick in the ass I needed to finally step out of my comfort zone and take control of my situation.*

CHAPTER 5

Change in an Instant

After Tom completely sideswiped me with this new information that I would be participating in the UBBT, I wanted to show him my appreciation (or lack thereof) and take him out to a nice dinner before he returned to California. As we all sat down, the waiter made his way over and asked for our drink order. I was the first to order and without any hesitation I blurted out, "I'll have a Coke."

As the waiter went around the table I started thinking about the leverage Tom had gotten on me so that I could not refuse his invitation to the UBBT. I continued to think how there had been many times in my life where I wanted to do something, but I could not get past the 'what ifs'. For the first time ever, I realized there was no longer anywhere to hide. In eighteen short months I would be standing in front of some of the most respected martial arts masters of our time and would either sink or swim. I knew that I couldn't keep hiding behind my façade with my insecurities and excuses, and finally admitted to myself that I was on a downward spiral that was sure to lead me towards a future filled with health problems, disappointment and regret. All this flashed through my mind while the waiter continued taking drink orders (and I subconsciously noted that Tom ordered a glass of water, not a soda). I thought to myself, 'How can I truly fulfill my promise to my son if I am not living up to my physical potential? Could it possibly be that this guy

Tom finally gave me the leverage I need to push myself into a healthier lifestyle altogether? Could it be that this is the start of a whole new me? Is it possible that, although I hate this man for embarrassing me in front of my entire student body, I secretly love him at the same time for challenging me to become more than what I am now?' As the waiter got to the last person, I made it a point to grab his attention. In a split second I was about to make a drastic change to my life.

"Waiter! Change my Coke to a water."

That decision to drink water rather than a soda was so much more than what it seemed at the time. I now realize that it was the broader decision to raise my standards and begin to make healthier choices that would carry me through the UBBT and beyond. You see, that day was about making a decision to completely rediscover myself and begin on a journey towards uncovering my true passion, meaning and purpose in life. I am proud to say that it is now ten years later and I have not even tasted a soda in all of that time, but what I am even more proud of is the list of other accomplishments that stemmed from that one decision to raise my standards and have water instead of soda.

Albert Einstein defined insanity as "doing the same thing over and over again and expecting different results". I finally realized that I would have to challenge my beliefs, change my habits and raise my standards if I were ever going to achieve my vision and fulfill my promises, and the first decision only took an instant to make. That decision to have water rather than Coke was the first decision that ultimately led me to not only discover my passion, but to align my beliefs and daily actions with what I valued the most.

CHAPTER 6

Overcoming the 'What Ifs'

Soon after Tom left, I took a fresh look at the test. I quickly realized that I couldn't jump right into it, but I had enough confidence in myself that if I broke the list down piece-by-piece and attacked it at my own pace, I would make some headway. The first bullet was 52,000 push-ups. If I broke that down into something more reasonable, I realized it was 1,000 per week, or less than 150 per day. Even more so, I could do six sets of 25 on my own time, which didn't seem all that bad. I moved on to the next bullet – 1,000 rounds of sparring, which I broke down into ten repetitions per day, two days per week. Then I did the same thing for sit-ups. With each bullet point I was able to check off my list, I felt my confidence slowly regaining itself. By no means was I out of the woods yet, but I was starting to make progress towards a new me.

Since I was at the karate school for most of my day, why not make the best of my time there? I decided to incorporate my workout within my classes and perform in front of my students. My biggest fear was trying something new in front of them, failing and never hearing the end of it. 'The guy on the magazine cover' shouldn't fail! The last thing I wanted to do was lose respect from my students considering the respect I had for myself at the time was quite low. I gathered up enough confidence to face my fear head on and made a commitment to start performing my form in front of my classes. As the time of my first performance approached I began to hear the voice in the back of my head – 'what if…' I began to feel a lump in my throat and butterflies in my stomach. 'What if I fall in the middle of the performance… what if I forget the movements… what if I freeze and embarrass myself?' I did battle with the 'what ifs', the lump and the butterflies, up to the last second. Every time I would begin to hear 'what if', I would consciously go into battle mode, taking control of my thoughts and replacing them with more positive words. 'I deserve this.' 'I worked hard for this.' 'I know I can do this because I have done this a thousand times before.' At this point the 'what ifs' were still there, but I had gathered up just enough confidence to push them back, take control and make it through the performance. Lo and behold, the exact opposite of what I expected occurred.

It was certainly not the best performance of my life. I lost balance a few times, my stomach was still hanging out over my belt and I certainly was not where I wanted to be, but something very encouraging happened. Every person in the room clapped and cheered for me. It seemed that they really appreciated the fact that I was stepping up and striving to set a better example. Because of that, it made me want to perform more often for my students who have looked up to me for many years. I immediately scheduled the next performance, then the next and then the next. With each performance my confidence increased, and with each increase in confidence my next performance improved and the crowd cheered louder. What they were not able to see is that the louder they cheered, the more they high-fived and the more they patted me on the back, the stronger I began to feel inside.

Before long the lump in my throat and the 'what ifs' began to show up less frequently. Tom had shown me the power of leverage, and I was starting to understand it and use it on myself. By scheduling my performances, putting myself out of my comfort zone, I obtained leverage on myself to force me to be constantly working towards my goals. It is very easy to tell yourself that you are going to put on a performance, or run in a marathon or any other goal you might want to attain – because if you back down, you can just make your excuses and hide behind your 'what ifs'; if you tell *other* people, people who you respect and whose opinions matter to you, then you have created leverage on yourself – you can't back out now, you *have* to do it, so you better work towards it and be ready for it! The more confident I became from each performance, the more people I would tell about the next performance, and the more I would work to top the previous one.

I saw the truth – for far too long, every time I had been faced with a challenge, I would take a step back into my comfort zone. Each time someone would ask me to join him or her for a run, a workout or some other activity I would take a step back. Each time my stomach would hurt, or I would feel the butterflies, I would take a step back. Every time I began to sweat because I was uncomfortable, I would take a step back. Finally I could see that each time someone put a challenge in front of me, I always took a step back. I had to make a commitment to myself that next time, instead of taking a step back I would take a step forward and confront the challenge. Once I implemented that plan, success after success, step after step, I began to grow my confidence, believe in myself and achieve my goals one by one. I was slowly beginning to think in terms of what would be possible if I continued to challenge my beliefs and stretch my limits.

STAGE 3

Achieve Your Goals

"It's not about the goal. It's about growing to become the person that can accomplish that goal."

– Anthony Robbins

CHAPTER 7

My Thermostat was Set at 72

Slowly but surely I was changing. All of the performances and practicing for them certainly began to have an impact on my waistline. Before long I was down to 205 pounds!

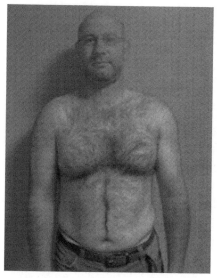

Me at 205 pounds... about this time, I felt like
I looked like everyone else around me

People who had not seen me in years could not help but comment. I was constantly getting positive reinforcement. "You look great!" "Keep it up!" "Wow, how did you do that?" The more people would comment, the better I would feel about myself. The better I felt about myself, the more I would perform and practice. The more I performed and practiced, the better I felt. I seemed to be caught in a fantastic chain of success. I began to realize that this was possible – my doubts and fears began to further lessen and I decided to raise my standards and really take it to the next level.

I made a commitment to myself that I would show up to the final test in the *best shape of my life*. I set a goal weight of 165 pounds for the final exam and began to weigh myself daily. I made the conscious decision to *step it up* and start working more diligently towards the attainment of my new goal. My energy and excitement level were at a peak. Soon I was working out several times a day. The scale started to move and I worked my way down to 195 pounds. The positive reinforcement continued to pour in. I kept taking on more and more. I performed every chance I could get; I did push-ups, sit-ups and ran with my students.

My beliefs were changing, but they weren't changing enough. It seemed that the minute the scale would hit 194 I began to put weight on again. Then when it hit 205 I began to take the weight off; the pats on the back, high-fives and congratulations would start again. I would work my way down to 194 then without fail I went right back up to 205 pounds and the cycle would repeat.

I remembered an analogy that I once heard comparing goal setting to the thermostat we all have in our homes. The thermostat is set at 72 degrees. When it gets too hot, the air conditioning turns on and cools the house to 72. When it gets cold, the heater kicks in to raise the temperature back to a comfortable 72 degrees. It seemed to me that my internal thermostat was set to around 200 pounds. The minute that my weight went to 205 I worked to bring it back down; when my weight would decrease to 194 I would relax, engage in old patterns and settle back to 200 pounds.

It was obvious that I was no longer 'the guy on the magazine cover'. I didn't look the same and more importantly I didn't need the façade anymore. I was more confident and was beginning to feel better about myself. I knew that if I was going to *take it to the next level* and actually be in the best shape of my life, I would no longer be able to settle for mediocrity and being "good enough". I would need to strive for excellence. I took a mental step to the side to reflect on the beliefs and actions that were getting me my current results to see which beliefs I could continue to challenge and change. I needed to reprogram my internal thermostat to 165 pounds!

CHAPTER 8

Could it be that I am just a Talking Dog?

I'm not sure why, but the high school lesson about Pavlov's dog has always stuck with me. We learned how Pavlov would feed his dog and ring a bell, and the dog would salivate. Every time he would feed the dog, he would ring the bell, conditioning the dog to associate the bell with food. Eventually he could ring the bell *without* feeding the dog but the dog would still salivate as if it was being fed. Pavlov showed that the ringing of the bell was ingrained deeply in the dog's subconscious. Was my brain really that different?

I dissected my day and took inventory of my actions. I quickly realized how many things I was doing daily as a matter of routine and habit that weren't benefiting my goals. It seemed that these routines were ingrained so deep in my subconscious that I was almost no longer in control, just like with Pavlov's dog. For example, I noticed that at the end of every day I would get home and "automatically" make my way over to the pantry where I would get a snack. Then I would retire to the couch where I would consume my snack until the first commercial break, at which point I would get up and get my *second* snack. Any time I would walk past the kitchen counter, I would pop a cookie into my mouth. I had been sabotaging myself, and I wasn't even aware of it until I sat down to take a serious look at my actions throughout the day. I realized at this point what my project would be for the next eighteen months. It was time to really get down to business.

If I was going to stick to my goal, I needed to do it with 100% commitment. The working out was easy and made me feel better about myself almost instantaneously – it was very immediate, positive feedback. The killer was going to be my diet. The day I left the hospital with my son I made a promise to myself that this was going to be the start of two new lives, and although my son was growing stronger and healthier, I hadn't really held up to my end of the bargain. I sought diet advice from friends, peers, nutritionists, books, the internet, anywhere and everywhere. What eventually enabled me to take my diet to the next level was when my friend, Dr. Nicholas Despotidis, made his own amazing physical transformation. I saw what he was able to accomplish and immediately knew – whatever he was doing, it was producing amazing results. I had to try it.

Day in and day out I stuck with my nutritional plan. I ignored temptations, no matter how inviting they seemed (and sometimes it was very difficult). I took the time to plan out my meals for the week so that I could never get to the point where I would have to go off-diet for the sake of eating whatever was convenient. Failing to plan is planning to fail. I started to see that I was slowly reaping the benefits from all my hard work. The weight was finally coming off and, more importantly, eating better made me *feel better* each and every day. Now it was clear to the naked eye that I was not only becoming stronger on the outside, but on the inside as well. My family, friends and students were impressed with my small accomplishments. It is important to mention that my confidence was growing and I was finally molding myself into the person I wanted to be. My goal was not just a farfetched vision – it was actually becoming a reality. Everyone around me respected the way I was pushing myself out of my own comfort zone to completely change my life for the better.

It has been said that the only thing that remains constant is change, and in my situation I couldn't agree more. My body and mind were going through unbelievable changes and my beliefs needed to follow the same pattern. My old beliefs had limited me to the shielded life I was living before my transformation began. I was chained to my old beliefs, but

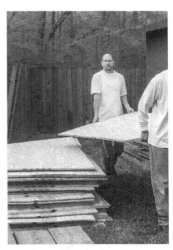

Alabama Home Build Project, 2005

it was now the perfect time to break the chains of my old patterns and set myself free. As the pounds were shedding, so was my old way of thinking. The "I can't do thats" and excuses were turning into "I cans" and determination. I traveled to Alabama to participate in a project to build a home for a man named Henry Lawson, who lost his home in a fire (and, surprisingly to anyone who knows me, managed to operate power tools without seriously injuring myself or anyone else). I went backpacking in the Sierra Nevada Mountains for a week with my UBBT team. I ran a half-marathon on the Las Vegas strip. I participated in a full-contact kickboxing match (and didn't lose any teeth). These are all things I would never have been able to accomplish with my old set of beliefs.

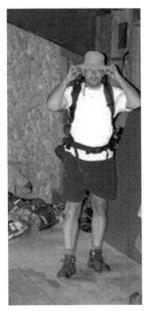

Sierra Nevada Hike, 2005

Over time, it became clear that the more I incorporated the things I was learning about exercise and nutrition into my everyday routine, the better results I achieved. Each pound of fat that I lost, and every compliment that I received, only reinforced my new beliefs. I now understood that eating nutritiously was not "insane", and I understood why my new beliefs made more sense. Every set of completed push-ups, every time the class cheered for me and every pat on the back reinforced a new belief that I was on the right path and well on my way to holding true to the promises I made to myself and my family.

We can "upgrade" our "programming" by replacing our old beliefs with new ones that better serve us, allowing us to lead lives of passion, purpose, fitness, health and fulfillment.

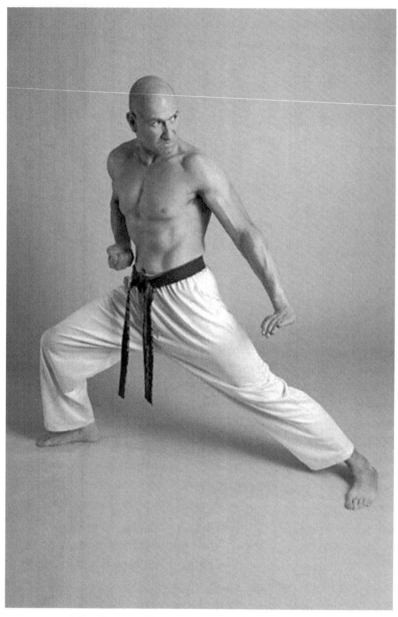

Me, after reaching my ideal weight of 165 pounds

STAGE 4

Inspire Others

"Learn and grow all you can; serve and befriend all you can; enrich and inspire all you can."

– William Arthur Ward

CHAPTER 9

Adding vs Subtracting

During my journey, I noticed some very interesting things. It seemed that the harder I would work, the harder most of the people around me would work also. Every day I would try to set the bar higher than the day prior and people around me caught light of that. If it stands true that every action has a reaction, then I believe that my positive motivation was also motivating others to set their bars a little higher. With this, it seemed that I attracted more positive people – people who shared the same passion, purpose and drive that I had newly developed. Similarly, because the people around me were more positive and inspiring people, I found myself being motivated to work harder to keep up with them.

Dr. Nicholas Despotidis has consistently been a source of this type of inspiration for me. Nick always seemed to be taking it one step beyond whatever I was achieving. During the time I was working on my personal transformation, Nick underwent his own as well – and went as far as entering a body building competition! And he won several awards – for his age group, for first time competitor and for overall competitor! I might host a business event, and it would be successful, but people weren't shocked by it – Nick would hold a business event and people would be blown away by what he accomplished. He always seemed to be able to reach a little bit further into excellence in everything he did. I saw the way he cycles himself through a clear goal-setting process, and the way he only surrounds himself with positive people who share his passion and dedication towards improvement. It was very galvanizing for me.

On the other side of the spectrum, I definitely noticed the crabs in the barrel of my life. As the proverb goes, if you put one crab in a barrel it will be able to climb out – but as soon as two or more crabs are in the barrel, any one crab that is trying to climb out will be pulled back down by the others. Some people might even be intentionally negative, but most of the time it is seemingly well-meaning people with the best intentions who are nevertheless trying to subconsciously sabotage you. They say things like, "It's no big deal; how can just one candy bar make a difference?" "You've lost too much weight, eat some ice cream!" "You've come such a long way, you deserve to treat yourself!" When you do something great, people are envious. Some people are able to take that envy and turn it into positive motivation – "if he can do it, *I can* do it!" Other people remain stuck on the negative – "if he can do it, *why can't I* do it?" People will either pull you into their world, or you will be strong enough to pull them into yours.

At one point, I was working closely in organization with some of my fellow martial arts school owners throughout New Jersey. During my time as 'the guy on the magazine cover', I was the leader of our organization for the business side of things, and my associates were de facto in charge of matters of our curriculum. As I progressed through my physical transformation, I began to take a more active role in our martial arts curriculum. I was doing a lot to broaden my knowledge, seeking out new styles and training with different masters, and I wanted to bring it back and share it with others – but this was received as stepping on peoples' toes. I was making changes, shaking up the status quo in pursuit of bigger and better things, seeking new ways to improve myself and to bring that improvement to my students and community, but some people are just resistant to change.

I realized that my colleagues liked me for who I was and that they were uncomfortable with the person I was becoming. They were comfortable with the overweight, soft Bryan Klein who was a business leader to them, but was not challenging to their training habits or their comfort zones. They liked the Bryan Klein who was complacent with mediocrity, and they felt threatened by the strong, confident individual I was becoming. The more I tried to take consistent action towards achieving my goals, the more they tried to pull me back to being the person *they* liked.

Misery definitely loves company – the negative people, even if it is unintentional, will seek to bring you down to their level to feel better about themselves. For me, it became about adding and subtracting – adding more, or spending more time around, positive people like Nick, and reducing the time I spent with the negative people. In some cases it meant eliminating some people from my life because, while I don't hold any ill-will towards them, they were the crabs unintentionally pulling me back down to where they felt comfortable. Rather than surrounding myself with people who held me back to keep me at a place they felt comfortable, I tried to surround myself with people who would pull me forward and help me to achieve my vision of a life of passion, productivity, happiness and excellence. I made the conscious decision to surround myself with **heroes** rather than **zeros**.

CHAPTER 10

Heroes and Zeros

Visualize two filing cabinets. One cabinet is marked "Possible", the other "Impossible". The people around you affect where you will file any given activity. When I first looked at it, the UBBT requirements were definitely filed under "Impossible", along with a lot of other things. As I surrounded myself with better quality people such as Nick, Tom and Alicia, I was slowly able to start moving things from the "Impossible" cabinet over to the "Possible" cabinet. I would actually imagine myself taking the file that said "52,000 push-ups" or "organize an environmental clean-up project", and moving it from one cabinet to the other. The more high-caliber people I surrounded myself with, the more things I saw as being "Possible" – this was nutrition for the mind. So I continued to seek out inspirational heroes. Sometimes it was a businessperson, sometimes a martial artist and sometimes it was just someone doing something great for his or her family. Sometimes I was able to actually meet these people in person, and sometimes I only knew them from their story on the internet or in their books, but in my mind even the people I could not meet were my close friends. I would cut out their pictures and post them on the wall of my office. I would read their books or read about them on the internet and watch their YouTube videos. For me, it was as if they were really there next to me pushing me along on my journey.

Nick Vujicic was one of the people who inspired me. His motto is "no arms, no legs, no worries". Nick was born without any limbs. For most of us, this would seem like an insurmountable challenge – even simple daily activities like brushing your teeth or combing your hair would be filed under "Impossible". Nick learned to overcome these obstacles and more. He has graduated college with a double major, started his own non-profit organization *Life Without Limbs* and leads a successful career as an inspirational and motivational speaker. At the age of 29 he has already done more with his life than most people will in twice as many years. More information about Nick can be found at *http://www. attitudeisaltitude.com*

Bethany Hamilton is another prime example of overcoming physical challenges. In 2003, at the age of 13, she was surfing in Hawaii when a tiger shark attacked her. She lost her left arm at the shoulder and 60% of her blood during the attack. Within just one month Bethany was back out on the water – she refused to let the ordeal deter her from her dream; a few years after that, she was able to realize her vision of becoming a professional surfer. Bethany is also an accomplished writer and public speaker, seeking to share her inspirational story of dedication, perseverance and triumph over adversity with millions of people. Bethany's website can be found at *http://bethanyhamilton.com*

Tom, one of my high-caliber friends you've already read about, is a leader in the martial arts community. He is known for his activism, his innovation and his passion. Aside from having created the Ultimate Black Belt Test, Tom also runs *The 100.*, "a martial arts business association for progressive, career martial arts school owners and teachers" which "designs substantive edu-

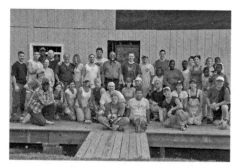

Tom Callos and me (back left), along with the rest of the UBBT Alabama House Build Team

cational curriculum for forward-thinking martial arts teachers involving peace education, bully prevention, dietary self-defense, anger management, environmental self-defense, community building, innovative black belt testing, art, writing, history, and character development." I could go on for days about Tom's résumé, all that he has accomplished in the world of professional martial arts and the many ways he's positively impacted my life. Tom can be reached through *http://tomcallos.com*.

It must take a special kind of instructor to produce a student who is as motivational and inspirational as Tom Callos. Tom's instructor is Master Ernie Reyes Sr., one of the most decorated and respected martial arts masters alive today. Master Reyes has been featured in virtually every national karate magazine in the world, has received numerous lifetime achievement awards and has starred along with his son in several full-length motion pictures. At 65 years old, he continues to run his school, his organization and his performance team, all of which are recognized as being among the best in the world. I have had the pleasure of meeting and talking with Master Reyes, of training with him and even of testing under him as a part of my quest to broaden my knowledge.

I used to look at the things these people would do and think to myself, 'I don't know how you do this.' I used to feel as if I were always coming up short. But I realized, the more I surrounded myself with these inspirational people, the greater the vision I had for myself was – and even if I were still falling a little short of what I had *hoped* to achieve, the things I *did* manage to accomplish were impressive. Constant and never-ending improvement became my overarching vision. And every time I would do something extraordinary, there would be someone behind me saying how I inspired them, which made me realize two things. First, the things I was accomplishing were in fact amazing even if they were not quite what I had set out to do; I had to stay focused on the positive of what I *was* able to do, not the negative of what I was unable to do. Second, I realized that I had become to other people what Nick and others had been to me. Through my transformation and achievements, I was inspiring the people around me.

STAGE 5

Create Your legacy

"Carve your name on hearts, not tombstones. A legacy is etched into the minds of others and the stories they share about you."

— Shannon Alder

CHAPTER 11

The Next level

I once read an essay titled "Mastery" by Stewart Emery. The first line read, "Mastery in our lives requires that we constantly produce results that go beyond the ordinary." Rather than just reading this essay I decided to commit it to memory, making it part of my daily life. Every morning I would read the words off of index cards that I created for myself. Each day I would commit another sentence of Stewart Emery's short essay to memory. I noticed with each day this essay was becoming much more than just words on a page. They were becoming part of my subconscious, they were helping to shape my beliefs and even more importantly, they were helping to shape my daily actions.

After completing my Ultimate Black Belt Test, I thought, 'What if I make my *own* UBBT to keep pushing myself to the next level?' I continued to create my own challenges to feed my body, mind and spirit the kind of things they needed to strengthen and grow. The year after that, I did it again, and again the next year and then again. I completely reinvented the curriculum at our martial arts school to be more in line with the new beliefs I had made and the new knowledge I had gained. Now, I am able to give back and offer the same kind of life-changing experiences I went through to my students through both UTA Martial Arts and THE MAX Challenge.

Back during the time I spent in New York while my wife was in NYU Medical Center for months, my staff at the martial arts school held a walk-a-thon for the March of Dimes, the organization that helped provide funding for Elijah's experimental surgery. The handful of people who participated raised a few thousand dollars. When I saw what just a few individuals were able to do, I thought to myself, 'What if *all* of my students got involved? How much money could we raise then? How much of an impact could we have on our community?' A year later, I held my first Martial Arts Extravaganza to benefit the March of Dimes. We raised over $32,000 in that first year, and our non-profit organization Martial Arts With Heart was born. Every year we fundraise for a different children's charity, culminating with our Martial Arts Extravaganza show. As of 2014, we are on our ninth year and have raised well over $500,000. While the money is definitely important to the charities, just as important is the awareness and activism that we are building with our students and our community.

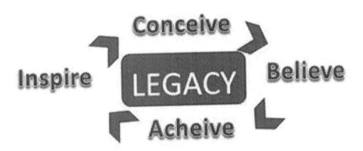

Every time I set out to do something new and extraordinary, from my full-contact kickboxing match, to the half-marathon in Las Vegas, to earning black belts in several other martial arts styles, I would cycle through the process again. I would conceive a new, expanded vision for my future. I would challenge my beliefs and seek to create new, more empowering beliefs. As I achieved each of these small victories, I saw that I was inspiring more people along the way. Every time I went through the process I became stronger on both the outside and the inside – I had developed a new habit of stepping up to beliefs instead of backing down.

I used that habit to create a new vision to share what I have learned with others and launched The MAX Challenge, a transformation program that combines fitness classes, success coaching and nutrition counseling. The changes that people began to make were nothing short of incredible. News of the success stories continued to spread. I am proud to say that in three short years The MAX Challenge has grown from an idea to just about 50 locations and over 10,000 participants. What I am most proud of is that "The MAX" is about much more then just physical transformations. It is a program that encourages others to step out of their comfort zones, discover their passions and achieve their dreams.

That is my legacy that I hope to leave behind for my children, students, community and world.

Want some more inspiration?
Go to www.TheMAXChallenge.com to hear inspirational success stories and learn more about THE MAX.

Your Story

The Transformation Epidemic

I want to thank you for having taken the time to read My Story. I hope you realize that it is not my intention to impress you with my achievements, but rather to *impress upon you* that change is possible. It does not come easy. It does not come overnight. The good news is that changing the way you look, the way you feel and most importantly changing your health is very possible and within your reach.

As possible as change is, it is also improbable for most Americans. Look at where we are heading as a society. Diabetes, heart disease, cancer and stroke are the biggest killers of Americans today. Yet, I have people still telling me every day that the way I eat and exercise is not sustainable. They tell me that it might be working now, but there's no way I will be able to do it day after day, year after year, or that it will continue to have the same results. How does that make any sense at all? Is it possible that, in the case of health, nutrition and fitness, the small minority has the right idea? How the heck could everyone else be wrong?

Think about this. If the way I am prescribing to eat or train is not sustainable, then I guess our current way of living *is* sustainable, right? Experts predict that the next generation of children will be the first generation that will not outlive their parents. If a shorter life span were not enough, science will miraculously extend the last few years of our lives with medicines and machines allowing us to live out our "golden years" in motorized chairs with oxygen tanks.

All of this and still we do not change!

As I mentioned earlier, Einstein said, "Insanity: doing the same thing over and over again and expecting different results." It seems that as a society we are all insane. Or could it be that there are invisible forces working against us? Before you dismiss the idea, think of it this way. Deep down inside we all know what needs to happen. We push it to the back of our minds, neatly tucked away into our subconscious. But back there, somewhere, we all know what we are doing when we eat fast food, sugary cereals and other processed foods.

We may decide at some point as individuals to change. We start off with the best of intentions. We might even join a gym. Then we go to lunch with our friends. "Come on, having only one can't possibly hurt you." "You will get back on track tomorrow." "Don't worry about it, you deserve it." Then there is the marketing: the McDonald's exactly where you need it at exactly the time you want it. It is not a mistake that there is a McDonald's on the corner you pass every morning, conveniently placed there for your morning coffee and egg sandwich. It is no mistake that there is a Burger King on the same block as your office just when you crave that quarter pounder. It is also no mistake that it looks, tastes and smells so damn good that you almost cannot say no.

All of these companies have spent countless hours and dollars in their laboratories creating the perfect burger, fries and soft drinks. The sole purpose of these companies is to produce a product that has just the right amount of crap in it, and it is marketed in such a way, that you cannot say no! You can't say no because, like Pavlov's dog, we have been conditioned to associate Happy with the word Meal. Their songs, pictures, smells and the combination of ingredients are designed with one intention – to get as many people as they can addicted to their product at the lowest cost possible. These companies would argue that we as Americans should exercise more self-control, that this is an issue of self-discipline, not of corporate responsibility. It sounds a lot like the argument they made a few years back for cigarettes.

Our society is on a train traveling 200 miles per hour towards a brick wall. We have the ability to stop this train wreck and change course, but first we have to realize that My Story is Your Story! My Story is the story of America and is quickly becoming the story of our world.

My vision is for each and every one of us to create new visions for living our own lives, the way we truly want to live, healthy, happy and full of energy to pursue our goals; each of us fueled by a clear and personal vision and mission. A vision based on a life of possibilities and passion. A vision and life's mission that is so compelling that it gives us the motivation to challenge our current beliefs and move in the direction of our dreams and goals! As each of us achieves our goals, we will inspire others to follow our lead and pursue their own individual dreams and goals.

They say that obesity is an epidemic. It has spread across America and the world like every other disease. From one person to the next, exponentially multiplying as it attacks individuals, families, communities, our country and our world. Let me dare to ask the question. Why can't the cure be an epidemic as well? Why can't we manufacture a movement that starts with you, changing you so drastically that you virtually become unrecognizable to your friends, family and those closest to you? A change that is so incredibly impressive that you are unrecognizable to even yourself! A change so extraordinary that it encourages all those around you to go to battle with their inner-most demons, to question their individual limitations and to commit to their own health and happiness.

Here is some more food for thought. Maybe this Obesity Epidemic is a gift that has been given to us as a society. Perhaps it is a challenge that has been set before us. Maybe this is a chance to pull together and overcome? As each and every one of us commits to living a life of health and happiness we break our bonds with the old way of eating. We consciously break the associations between happiness and (junk) food.

Pavlov's dog is cursed for the rest of his life. Every time someone rings that damn bell, he salivates and craves food! The curse is that the dog does not have the awareness to break that conditioning. We have the ability to stop and think about why we are making the choices we make. Are they our own choices? Are they the choices that will lead us to where we want to be? Do our actions support our visions? Or are we living out someone else's story? Could it be that by breaking this bond, we become aware of all the other stories that have been sold to us? Is there something else to life? Could this be our path to freedom?

I encourage you to not only turn to the next page in this book, but to turn to the next chapter in your life. As you turn this page, I hope that you open your mind and heart and fully engage in this process. My greatest wish is that you discover your passion and life's vision for a whole new world of possibilities.

STAGE 1

Conceive Your Vision

"Be daring, be different, be impractical, be anything that will assert integrity of purpose and imaginative vision against the play-it-safers, the creatures of the commonplace, the slaves of the ordinary."

— Cecil Beaton

CHAPTER 12

Making It About YOU

Remember this picture from the beginning of My Story?

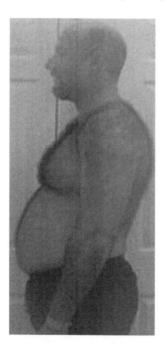

Please take a moment to look at the picture above. (Don't take too long or the horror of it may burn a permanent hole in your retina!) As you look at the picture, think about the words that you would use to describe this person. Do you think this person is strong and powerful? Does this person have high energy? Leadership qualities? Do the words health and fitness pop into your mind? Does this person have the energy to take consistent daily action towards his goals? Use the space below to write down the first few descriptive words that pop into your mind when you look at the picture above.

_____

_____

_____

What activities do you think this person engages in regularly? Sitting on the couch? Watching television? Daily exercise? Running long distances? Full contact martial arts? – or – Running to the refrigerator and full contact snacking? (Let's continue with the exercise and make a short list of the activities you think this person engages in daily.)

_____

_____

_____

Let's take some time to examine this person's beliefs? Would you say that his belief system is strong and empowering or limiting and restrictive? Do you think that he believes, "My body is a temple" and "Garbage in, garbage out" or maybe it is more like "Live for today and don't worry about tomorrow?"

_____

_____

_____

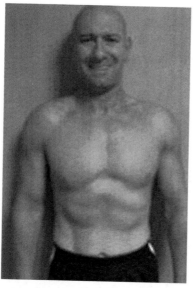

Let's repeat the exercise again, this time focusing on the picture above. How do you think the guy in the picture feels about himself? Is he strong and confident? Does he have high energy? Tell me, does he look lazy or productive? (Record the first few words that pop into your mind to describe the person above.)

_____

_____

_____

What beliefs do you think this person has? How does he view the world? Are his beliefs empowering or limiting? Does he believe his body is a temple – or – live for today and don't bother with tomorrow?

_____

_____

_____

What activities do you think this person engages in daily? Fitness, sports, full-contact martial arts – or professional eating, taste testing and TV-watching?

_____

_____

_____

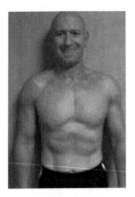

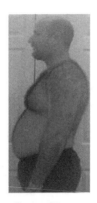

Fit Picture   *Scary Picture*

In case you did not realize it, both of those pictures are of the same person, and that person is me! The amazing thing is that those pictures were taken just about a year apart.

Look at these pictures one more time next to each other.

Stop for a minute and really appreciate what has been accomplished here. Take a few seconds to recognize the emotional, spiritual and physical transformation that took place in a relatively short amount of time. Don't only recognize the more obvious physical change but visualize the inner changes that took place. Please go back to that first picture a few pages back. Look at the descriptive words, the beliefs and daily actions you listed on the bottom of the page and rewrite them in the space provided under the "scary" picture on this page. Now do the same for the "fit" picture.

The point I am trying to make is that the most obvious changes I made were on the outside but the most important ones took place on the inside.

Now it is your chance to create your own transformation. This is your opportunity to make a promise to yourself, your family, your community and your world!

This section of the book is no longer about me. In this section we will take a journey towards creating your vision, developing the beliefs to support you in the achievement of that vision, set and achieve your goals and develop your plan for inspiring others.

I look forward towards your success!

CHAPTER 13

Identifying Your Values

To *conceive your vision* sounds like such a simple thing. Know what you want. Everybody knows what he or she wants, right? Of course we do! I want to be perfectly healthy. I want to have a lot of money. I want to have a happy family. How hard can it be to know what you want? The problem that arises is that we oftentimes have conflicting desires. I want to be perfectly healthy, but I also want to eat pizza and drink beer while watching the game on Sunday. I want to have a lot of money, but I want to be on vacation all the time, not spend my life working. I want to have a happy family, but I want to spend time watching television, out with my friends and doing things for myself.

The challenge is in identifying your values and finding out which of them is most important to you. If having a piece of cake every day is more important than your own health and your ability to live a long life, and to consistently be around for your children and family, then that is your choice. However, I don't think you would still be reading this if that were the case. I think that most of us will agree that our long-term goal of health and fitness ranks much higher than the short-term taste of any food. But are you acting in a way that aligns with those values?

It is important to make the conscious realization that you cannot have your cake and eat it, too. You cannot have the long-term health and fitness that you envision for yourself without giving up those short-term pleasures of poor food choices and poor exercise habits. No matter what you might see on the late-night infomercials about how you can lose weight while eating all of your favorite foods – it just isn't true. (Don't fear! When you change your diet to make healthier choices, you will be pleasantly surprised to find that good foods are delicious as well!) One of the most important benefits to acting in line with your values is the happiness you gain. Think about how you feel when you intend to lose weight but eat a big piece of chocolate cake, or when you intend to save money but buy a new car with a hefty monthly payment. Frustrated. Negative. Disappointed.

It's time to give up those conflicting values and focus on your real vision for yourself. Take a moment to consider what some of your highest values are. Write them in the space provided on the next page. I will even help you get started with your first one.

1. Your LIFE

2.

3.

4.

5.

6.

Now, you may be wondering why I filled in the number one spot on *your* values list for you. It's very simple – none of the rest of your list will have any meaning without that first value. It doesn't matter what was on your list, if there is no *you* then you cannot value it. Even if you didn't realize this right away, I think you at least implicitly understand the general idea because you are still here reading this!

My intention with this book is to help motivate you to make the changes you want to improve the quality of your life. By improving the quality of your life, you will be in a better position to affect and appreciate the rest of your values. Things that positively impact your health improve your life, which in turn enables you to achieve the rest of your values. We state this by saying, 'When we have *energy*, we can take *action*. When we take *action*, we achieve our *goals*.'

Your goals should be SMART goals. The SMART principle is a common management tool that has been invaluable to me over the years in sports, business and life. It stands for

- Specific
- Measurable
- Attainable
- Relevant
- Timely

Go back to your mind map. Identify four SMART goals you have for yourself to accomplish during your 10-week transformation. Write them down on the next page. Then, on the following page, attempt to describe how each of those specific goals relates back to the values you listed earlier.

What four specific SMART goals do you want to accomplish during your 10-week transformation?

1.

2.

3.

4.

How do your four goals relate back to your values? How will achieving each goal improve the quality of your life?

1.

2.

3.

4.

CHAPTER 14

The Promise

By now I hope you have begun to recognize the possibilities. You absolutely can make relatively quick and lasting changes to your health, fitness and appearance. You have already recognized the desire to change within yourself. In fact, you are probably very familiar with those feelings. Those are the feelings that have surfaced every time that you start towards your vision. But why have you never succeeded in achieving that vision? What is going to be different this time?

This time, we are going to turn that tiny spark of motivation into a burning inferno, and it starts with the creation of your vision. *You must create a vision that is powerful enough to keep you going through the tough times.* Those times when you could really use a cookie or a beer after a long day at work. Those times when your muscles are sore and aching and you would rather stay in bed than drag yourself to your workout. Your vision will become your personal guidance system that will keep you on track – minute-by-minute, day-by-day, week-by-week and month-by-month. Every decision must be measured through the filter of your long-term vision, allowing you to take consistent daily action towards its attainment. In short, this must be your turning point. Just like that moment, minutes before my son was born, when I made that promise to be the best example I could be for my family and karate students. This is your moment.

STAGE 2

Challenge Your Beliefs

"If you don't change your beliefs, your life will be like this forever. Is that good news?"

– W. Somerset Maugham

CHAPTER 15

Invisible Fences

Farmers today are able to utilize an amazing technology with their horses and other animals. They no longer need fences large enough to physically keep the animals caged in. Today, they use thin wires strung between fence posts that are slightly electrified. The animals learn very quickly that touching the fence leads to a shock – similar to how Pavlov's dog was taught that the sound of the bell meant food. However, the animals don't actually understand that it is the wire that makes the shock when touched. They just know where they cannot walk. With this, even if the fence breaks, or is later removed, the animals will not attempt to cross the invisible line that they associate with that small electric shock.

People, in their own minds, are just like those animals in the field. Everyone has his or her invisible fences. Humanity as a whole has plenty of invisible fences. If we just accept that they are really there and never challenge the idea, never approach the area where the fence is because we are afraid of that shock, we limit what we are capable of.

Think of some things that people KNEW to be true, and didn't even bother to challenge. What things did people just KNOW were impossible, but are now possible? For the majority of human history, everyone KNEW that the world was flat until someone challenged that belief and sailed around it. For the majority of human history, everyone KNEW that traveling to the moon was impossible until people challenged that belief and flew there in what amounted to a giant aluminum can with less computing power than the average smartphone owner carries in his or her pocket today.

For decades, the four-minute mile was considered something of the Holy Grail of track and field. Running a mile in under four minutes was something no one had ever accomplished yet in the early 1950s. While the record had slowly approached it in the preceding decades, it seemed to have stagnated at a second and a half away from the magical invisible fence of four minutes, and stayed that way for nine years until May 6, 1954, when Roger Bannister completed the mile run in 3 minutes 59.4 seconds. Forty-six days later, John Landy beat Bannister's record. By 1964, Jim Ryun was able to beat the four-minute mile as a *high school junior*. Today, many runners break the four-minute barrier on a regular basis. The world record is currently 3 minutes and 43 seconds – over *17 seconds* faster than people even believed was possible.

Identify some beliefs you have currently filed under "impossible" that really should be moved to your "possible" folder. Write them down on the next page. An example of this exercise:

1. I can't get up at 4:30 am to train before work.

2. I can't give up my hot cheesesteaks and cold beer after a long day at work.

3. I haven't worked out in a year/5 years/ever, I won't be able to keep up with the class.

4. I can't stay compliant with my nutrition while I'm at work all day/ busy taking care of my kids all day.

5. I can't possibly run a half-marathon/mud run/5K/around the block.

6. I can't get in the best shape of my life at my age. There's no way I can be as fit now as I was at 25.

List your "impossible" beliefs that are actually very possible.

1.

2.

3.

4.

5.

6.

Now cross them all out!

CHAPTER 16

Reassess and Rewrite

You already recognize that the beliefs you listed, while they seem impossible now, truly are not. But what leads you to believe these things are impossible in the first place? All of your beliefs are held up and validated by information and other beliefs.

People used to think the world was flat. Why? Well, all the smartest people, the people who knew what they were talking about, believed it was flat. "Everyone I know believes the world is flat." "My cousin's friend's brother is a sailor, and he sailed all the way to the edge and he saw it, so it's obviously flat." None of these change the truth, and once people were willing to challenge the belief they were able to identify more facts and develop new, more accurate beliefs.

Lots of people assume that visible, "six-pack" abdominal muscles are purely genetic. Why? Well, "my brother has abs and he eats whatever he wants and doesn't work out that hard." "I've tried to get abs before and I wasn't able to do it." "My best friend's roommate's uncle read somewhere that abs are genetic and that it doesn't matter what you eat or how hard you train." The truth is that, like with most things with your body, genetics and conditioning each play a role – and anyone willing to challenge the belief that they *can't*, and really go after their goal, will be able to develop new, better beliefs. We need to challenge our beliefs from the ground up.

On the next page you will rewrite one of your SMART goals from Stage One. The more times you write it, and the more times you read it, the more power you gain from it and the more likely you will be to achieve your vision. (We will be expanding on this exercise later and repeating it for *all* of your SMART goals.)

Then, you will complete the following sentence three times – "I believe I can't because…"

Finally, you will complete *this* sentence three times – "I believe I **can** because…"

Goal:

I believe I can't because...

I believe I can't because...

I believe I can't because...

Now physically cross out all the negative things you just wrote.
I believe I **can** because...

I believe I **can** because...

I believe I **can** because...

STAGE 3

Achieve Your Goals

"All men dream, but not equally. Those who dream by night in the dusty recesses of their minds, wake in the day to find that it was vanity; but the dreamers of the day are dangerous men, for they may act on their dreams with open eyes, to make them possible."

– T. E. Lawrence

CHAPTER 17

Breaking Out of the Rut

Now that you are willing to challenge your beliefs, you need to take *action* if you want to achieve your *goals*. But what action are you going to take? You need to identify patterns of behavior that you are trapped in, so that you can change those behaviors. Pavlov's dog was cursed – every time someone rang the bell, he would salivate uncontrollably. What bells are ringing in your life making you salivate?

Next time you reach for an Oreo – Stop. Put the cookie down. Assess. Do you really want that cookie? Is it really worth it? Is it really in line with your values? Or is it just a response to a ringing bell? Redirect. Throw the cookie away. Grab an apple. Grab a salad. Throw the entire jar of cookies away. Fill it with fruit.

Any time you find yourself falling into a negative pattern, you need to make the conscious effort to stop yourself and step out of the situation. Once you have taken a step back you can really look at the actions you are taking and decide if they are in line with your goals. Stop. Assess. Redirect. For me, as I mentioned earlier in this book, it was the habit of getting home from work, grabbing a snack from the junk-food cabinet and plopping down onto the couch to watch television (and then a second snack during the commercials), like clockwork every night. Stopping was the hardest part. Once I stopped myself and assessed what I was doing, I saw that I wasn't even that hungry – it was just the habit of the activity. The television was for me what the bell was for Pavlov's dog. Time to sit down and relax? Grab a snack before I do. Commercial? Sure, it's about time for another snack (how convenient). Did I even really need to sit down and watch television? What was I watching? The same as what I was eating – garbage. How many better things could I be spending my time on – something for work, or just spending time with my family after a busy day. Stop. Assess. Redirect.

On the next pages, identify four patterns that you find yourself falling into that need to be broken for you to achieve the vision you have developed for yourself. For each of these patterns, think of three ways to redirect yourself. I've provided my example below:

Pattern: Get home from work, grab a snack, sit on couch and watch television. Potential for more snacks.

Redirect: Get home from work, take out laptop or magazine and read up on new training concepts or research in health and fitness.

Redirect: Get home from work, talk to wife, play with kids, pet cat.

Redirect: Get home from work, relax listening to music or meditating. Unwind.

Pattern:

Redirect:

Redirect:

Redirect:

Pattern:

Redirect:

Redirect:

Redirect:

Pattern:

Redirect:

Redirect:

Redirect:

Pattern:

Redirect:

Redirect:

Redirect:

Here I have provided some ideas for activities that you can use to replace your negative patterns. Feel free to add any activities to this list that are in line with your values.

– Sit down and relax. Just relax. Take three minutes for yourself.
– Read the paper or a book. (Hey! You are doing that right now!)
– Listen to music.
– Meditate.
– Spend time with your significant other.
– Spend time with your children/pets/family.
– Catch up on or get ahead with some work.
– Stretch for 5 minutes.
– Go for a run/perform a light workout.
– Plan out your meals for the week.
– Cook your meals for the week.

CHAPTER 18

Take Action... NOW!

There is a famous quote by Napoleon Hill, the father of the modern self-help genre, which says, "Every failure brings with it the seed of an equivalent success." I think a better quote would be that every *success* brings with it the seed of an *even greater success*. When you take consistent daily action, you *will* achieve your goals. Every day, every small action, even the seemingly meaningless things we do throughout our day – everything adds up either to our success or our failure.

Remember Stewart Emery's essay I talked about before?

Through applying the principles in his essay I realized that getting by isn't enough – if you are looking to get by, you are sliding backwards away from your goals. I learned that there is no standing still, there are only two directions; forwards or backwards. Essentially I learned to dedicate myself to excellence, surround myself with things that represented excellence and to expect the best from myself.

All of our little actions add up. There are a few french fries left on your child's plate... do you pop them in your mouth? You know there are 23 almonds in a serving... do you count them out, or just grab a handful? You go out after work on a Tuesday night with some co-workers... do you have that one beer to unwind, or do you order a glass of water? They share some bar snacks... do you finish off their last mozzarella stick and buffalo wing, or do you decline? Every small action that is in line with your values is a small achievement. Each small achievement adds power and substance to the new belief structure that you are building for yourself. As that new belief system becomes stronger, that next small victory becomes that much easier – saying no to those three french fries or that last mozzarella stick will be hard the first time, but it will be easier the second time, the third time and every time after that. The flip side is also true – saying yes to those french fries or that mozzarella stick this time will make it easier to say yes next time. Don't allow yourself to compromise. Know what you want. Know what action you need to take to get it. Don't allow anything to get in your way.

There are two exercises for this chapter. One of them is a long-term exercise called the Chain of Success. The Chain of Success is how you will measure your attendance, or your adherence to your workout schedule, as well as your compliance with nutrition. Every day. "What? That's crazy talk! That's not possible! That's not sustainable! I can't keep that up every day!" All right, maybe that wasn't your initial reaction – maybe you've already taken enough away from this book to know better. But either way, think about what would support those beliefs in someone? The idea for the Chain of Success is simple. You will start with a calendar. Every day that you stay compliant with your nutrition, you will put a line from the top left to the bottom right. Every day that you complete your workout, you will put a line from the top right to the bottom left, forming an 'X'. When you do it the next day and put two 'X's next to each other, then the next day and the next, you will start to see the chain developing.

How do you think you will feel when you have a chain 70 'X's long on your calendar as a testament to your vision? Proud. Confident. Unstoppable! When I would compete in martial arts tournaments, I would do a lot of things to build my confidence. I took a picture of myself and wrote in big letters on it, "CHAMPION", and pinned it to the ceiling above my bed. As I lay in bed at night I would listen to meditation tapes and look up at that picture. When I woke up, it was the first thing I saw. And I would mark off my training days on the calendar with big 'X's. I would be completely confident going into the competition because I knew that I had more 'X's on my calendar than anyone else. That's the feeling I want you to get from the Chain of Success. Don't allow yourself to compromise. Little things will get in the way. Life happens. There are a million excuses for why you could miss a day and have a break in your Chain. Don't break the Chain.

For the other exercise for this chapter, we are going to be rewriting our goals and beliefs again as we did in Chapter 16, but we will add an extra sentence: "The action I'm going to take is..." Remember, the more we write and read our SMART goals, the more power we gain from them and the more likely we are to achieve those goals.

Goal:

I believe I can't because...

I believe I can't because...

I believe I can't because...

Now physically cross out all the negative things you just wrote.
I believe I **can** because...

I believe I **can** because...

I believe I **can** because...

The action I'm going to take is...

Goal:

I believe I can't because...

I believe I can't because...

I believe I can't because...

Now physically cross out all the negative things you just wrote.
I believe I **can** because...

I believe I **can** because...

I believe I **can** because...

The action I'm going to take is...

Goal:

I believe I can't because...

I believe I can't because...

I believe I can't because...

Now physically cross out all the negative things you just wrote.
I believe I **can** because...

I believe I **can** because...

I believe I **can** because...

The action I'm going to take is...

Goal:

I believe I can't because...

I believe I can't because...

I believe I can't because...

Now physically cross out all the negative things you just wrote.
I believe I **can** because...

I believe I **can** because...

I believe I **can** because...

The action I'm going to take is...

STAGE 4

Inspire Others through Your Accomplishments

"Good actions give strength to ourselves and inspire good actions in others."

— Plato

CHAPTER 19

Plan for Success

I mentioned earlier in this book the story about the crabs in the barrel. What I want you to consider now is this – who are the crabs in your barrel?

Remember, these people are most likely not maliciously trying to sabotage you. They probably have only good intentions if they are people who care about you, but it is important to be able to recognize poor advice and have a plan to deal with it before it comes up.

Consider this situation. You are out to dinner with friends. You order a nice, compliant dinner – steak, side of vegetables, making sure nothing is cooked in butter, water to drink. Your friends look at you funny as you are giving your specifications to the server. Dessert time comes. Your friends order cheesecake and pie. You order a black coffee. How does everyone at the table react? "Come on, have a piece of cake." "You deserve it." "You work out so much, it counteracts the cake!" "You didn't even order anything good for dinner, and now you aren't having dessert?"

When I would walk by the pizza parlor in the shopping center where my martial arts school used to be located, the pizza guy would say to me, "You haven't been in for a while," to try to make me feel guilty. "You do all that working out, you will burn it off anyway."

Maybe your friends wouldn't say something like that. Maybe they are supportive and know how hard you are working towards your goals. But I'm sure you can think of someone in your life – a friend, family member or co-worker – who would say something to that effect. I'm not saying that you have to get rid of these people completely or cut them out of your life – if anything, I want you to try to turn them from a problem into an opportunity. What I am saying is that you need to consciously develop a strategy for dealing with these situations *before* they come up. Because you know they will come up, and just as with your nutrition, failing to plan is planning to fail.

On the next page, I want you to identify three of the crabs in your barrel For each one, I want you to think of something they would say that might sabotage you, and then consider how you will respond to them.

Person:
Potential Negative Statement:

Planned Response:

Person:
Potential Negative Statement:

Planned Response:

Person:
Potential Negative Statement:

Planned Response:

CHAPTER 20

Identify Your Heroes

Even more important than limiting the influence of the negative people around you and the amount of time you spend with them is maximizing your access to and time spent with heroes and positive people. The three people you associate with the most are the three people you will be most influenced by. Surround yourself with people who will support you in your efforts to achieve your vision.

I already told you about my heroes. Some of them are friends from my personal life or people that I have been fortunate enough to meet. Some of them I have yet to meet in person – but they are still heroes of mine, and their stories, accomplishments and message were still influential to me. I want you to identify three people who are already in your life or who you have the possibility of meeting and spending time with. List them. Make an effort to spend more time with them and less with the crabs in your life. Then, list three people who you can "study from afar" – people you might never meet but who still serve as a source of inspiration for you.

Local Heroes:

1.

2.

3.

Global Heroes:
1.

2.

3.

    As you are seeking inspiration from these people, before long you will find that **you** have become the source of inspiration for the people around you. They will want to know what you are doing to get the results you are getting. "Where are you going to work out?" "What are you eating?" "How do you do it? The transformation is incredible!" All the praise should only serve to motivate you even more. It becomes the ultimate leverage you can have over yourself – you have all these people who are now inspired by **you**! You don't want to let them down, so you keep pushing hard knowing that it will help the people around you. You develop a virtuous cycle – you inspire those around you, and knowing how much of a positive influence you are for other people inspires you!

STAGE 5

Create Your Legacy

"Accept the challenges, so you may feel the exhilaration of victory."

– General George Patton

CHAPTER 21

Your Next level

As you continue to make progress in your transformation and find inspiration from those around you in your life, I'm sure you'll find that you, too, cannot just leave well enough alone. You'll have more energy, providing you with the ability to take action and achieve your goals. As you've learned, I'm not talking about a commitment to just "get by", because that will only take you farther from your goals. I'm talking about a commitment towards mastery, a commitment to *excel* or an *extreme commitment to do the extraordinary*. Through this **massive action** you'll ask some new, more positive 'what ifs' of yourself and accomplish things you never thought imaginable.

Throughout life, you always have the choice to settle or to continue to create your own challenges that feed your body, mind and spirit. With every small victory, you'll find that you're inspiring others as you became stronger on the outside and the inside. Isn't that exactly the legacy of yourself that you hope to leave behind in the world?

Push yourself to take your life to the next level. Write down three goals that you have already accomplished, how you can take that goal to the next level and the actions you can perform to accomplish your new goals. And see what you can do!

Accomplished goal:
Next-level goal:
Next-level actions:

Accomplished goal:
Next-level goal:
Next-level actions:

Accomplished goal:
Next-level goal:
Next-level actions:

Are you feeling intimidated? Don't be! You've already challenged your beliefs and created new patterns. You have a support network and you understand how to surround yourself with positive people who will help you accomplish your goals. As you develop a transformation cycle, you'll inspire those around you and they, in turn, will serve to continually inspire you!

Center of the Universe

We are all taught about how everything revolves around the sun. After all, without the sun there would be no life! As true as this is, I think there is a new possibility lying at the center of the entire universe. What if we each adopted a new truth? What if, tomorrow, scientists announced a new and exciting breakthrough discovery that at the center of the universe there was a previously undiscovered and mysterious source of power and inspiration – YOU!

Some of us may still hold this not to be true. Some of us may be thinking, 'how @*$&ing selfish is this guy to put himself and ask us to put ourselves first? My kids are more important to me, my family is more important to me and I have to sacrifice in order to give to them.'

Ask yourself these questions: If you are not here to experience yourself, your family, your friends and your world, then do those things exist for you? How can you sacrifice to give to your children if you aren't around to have anything to give?

What is even worse is being here with them, today, living a life void of excellence, health and purpose. The most contagious and life-threatening epidemic we face is mediocrity. What I have come to discover is that my weight was only a reflection of what was going on inside of me; all of the disharmony, unsatisfied dreams and misguided ambitions manifested themselves in the outward appearance of my body. This project was just a way for me to identify and then feed my true passions in life. Like peeling back the layers of an onion, slowly but surely I am discovering what makes me the most happy and fulfilled, and where my true passions and life purpose lie.

The thing that has surprised me the most is that the more I focus on improving and discovering myself, the brighter I shine in the world. Energy grows from within and is the source of life for everything around it. The brighter your energy shines, the brighter everything around you shines as well. In other words – the more confidence, joy, health and purpose I experience, the more positive the influence on those around me. Isn't that the greatest gift I can give to myself, my family, my friends and ultimately my world?

So back to the question from the beginning of this book – why did I do it? I did it to change my body. Then I realized I did it to change my mind. Ultimately, I'm doing it to change the world and take it all to THE MAX!

The End...

- or -

The Beginning...

The choice is yours!

Change your life with THE MAX!

As you know, THE MAX Challenge is not a gym and it's not some fad diet. It's a 10-week life-altering fitness and nutrition program with the power to transform lives.

To watch videos of real member stories or begin your journey with THE MAX, visit **themaxchallenge.com**.

Interested in bringing THE MAX to your neighborhood? Learn about franchising opportunities at maxfitfranchising.com.

Made in the USA
Middletown, DE
20 July 2015